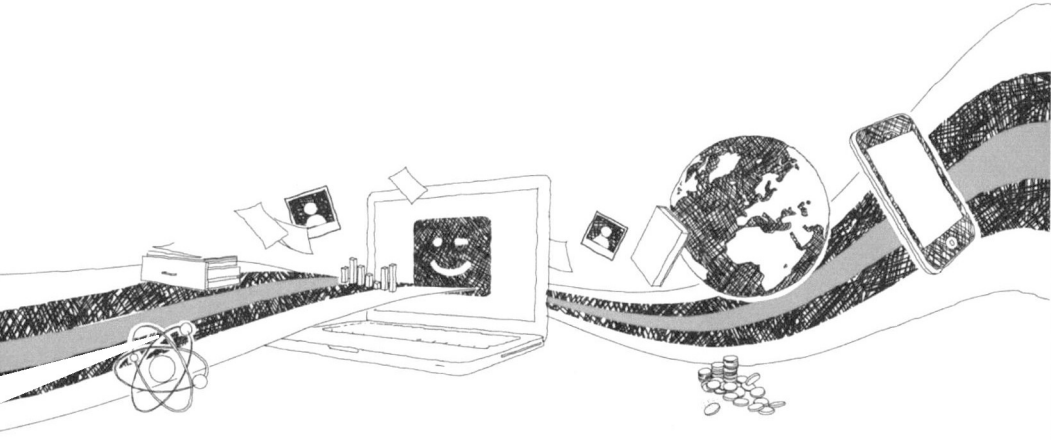
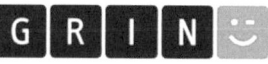

Bibliographic information published by the German National Library:

The German National Library lists this publication in the National Bibliography; detailed bibliographic data are available on the Internet at http://dnb.dnb.de .

Imprint:

Copyright © 2015 GRIN Verlag, Open Publishing GmbH
Print and binding: Books on Demand GmbH, Norderstedt Germany
ISBN: 978-3-668-04688-7

This book at GRIN:

http://www.grin.com/en/e-book/304220/mdma-case-study-a-case-for-decriminaliza-tion-or-prohibition

Alexander Syder

MDMA Case Study. A Case for Decriminalization or Prohibition?

GRIN Publishing

GRIN - Your knowledge has value

Since its foundation in 1998, GRIN has specialized in publishing academic texts by students, college teachers and other academics as e-book and printed book. The website www.grin.com is an ideal platform for presenting term papers, final papers, scientific essays, dissertations and specialist books.

Visit us on the internet:

http://www.grin.com/

http://www.facebook.com/grincom

http://www.twitter.com/grin_com

MDMA: significance of effects and future scientific investigation

MDMA has become one of the most popular, recreational drugs in the westernized world (Parrott et al, 2001). Although the use of MDMA has become increasingly widespread, there exists a serious debate amongst the psychiatric researchers as to whether MDMA (ecstasy) is a potentially dangerous and lethal drug to the individual using the substance (Mohamed et al, 2011; Parrott, 2013a, 2014). There is however an opposing argument amongst a group of researchers that MDMA has therapeutic benefits that can be used for self-healing, alleviating social anxiety and problems with social integration in a psychotherapeutic environment (Greer and Tolbert, 1986; Sessa and Nutt, 2007). The media and state politicians in western countries have however been pursuing a discourse of promoting MDMA as the same status as cocaine and heroin, with the same psychological and physiological properties; the reason is partially political with the populist stance of political parties to be seen as tough on drugs, often referred to as the 'War on Drugs' coined by President Nixon in 1971 (Smith, 2007). There is a divide therefore on the issue of MDMA as to whether this is a debate on the nature of the drug and its effects. Studies have been aimed at defining ecstasy from a premise of whether the effects are bad or good, studies leaning towards one of the observations typically rather than allowing for equal debate; the research can become political as opposed to unbiased scientific research, as Meyer's (2013) argues research into ecstasy has come from its most vociferous detractors and the most ardent supporters. The studies of beneficial effects are nonetheless increasingly limited, with little opportunity to test this proposed hypothesis. For instance in the US, the DEA has categorized MDMA as a Schedule 1 drug, a drug that through its classification is considered incredibly dangerous with high federal penalties for the possession and supply of the drug. This has limited the progression of medical and psychiatric research into the properties of MDMA; particularly the positive properties which require further longitudinal studies into the effects of MDMA (Sessa and Nutt, 2007; Smith, 2007; Mithoefer, 2011; Caulkins et al, 2014).

The legacy of this prohibitionist movement of MDMA and many other illicit substances stems from the United States under President Nixon in 1971 who declared a 'war on drugs' (Guardian, 2015). Over £1 trillion has been spent across society in order to eradicate drugs but to no fruition; instead the criminal market and black market of drugs continues to grow and bring in billions of pounds for criminal syndicates and gangs (Caulkins et al, 2014). The case for decriminalization merits serious discussion and warrants as a viable option of UK drug policy in the future. The existing model of criminalization has clearly not worked to tackle the issue of substance abuse, with higher levels of demand and the recent growth of legal highs; the main proposition of criminalization is that it deters those though legal punitive policies, however, there is increasing evidence that criminalization has not deterred those from using illicit drugs (Ward, 2013). The case for legal measures has been applied throughout America and spread to the UK in a populist, conservative approach to drug use with criminalization measures and moral panics spread throughout the media portraying a society addicted to drugs (Sessa and Nutt, 2007). Education of drugs, rather than legality should be applied in understanding and tackling substance abuse (Ward, 2013). The historical conception of MDMA is therefore an important premise upon which to investigate the effects of MDMA on the individual and society across the past several decades. MDMA or more popularly known as 'ecstasy' began a huge up-rise in popular consumption during the 1980s and late 1990s in Britain. The drug grew in Texas with the late night-life, club scene but took of massively in Britain in the late 90s with the rave techno music scene establishing a large base of popularity with the young (Agar et al, 2004). The approach by the government in the US was followed thereafter in the UK. It is important to note that during the 80s and 90s Britain, particularly under Tony Blair's administration drew heavy influence from US policy in areas of criminological significance; Tony Blair wished to emulate the example of the New Democrats under Bill Clinton. The prohibitionist approach launched in the 1970s by President Nixon has continued to spread to UK drug policy. However, there exists a serious debate as to whether MDMA should be in the same classification as heroin and cocaine, two highly addictive drugs with observable negative and devastating effects on those who abuse the substances. Furthermore Professor David Nutt has argued against the hypocrisy of the criminalization of MDMA whilst the most dangerous drug, and costly drug, alcohol remains legal alongside tobacco (Sessa and Nutt, 2007). It is important to note that in the past MDMA was suggested and promoted as a form of therapeutic enhancement for therapists to offer and suggest for patients with unresolved social issues, relationship problems and social anxiety (Griffin, 2012). The original suggestion was made by Dr. Alexander T. Shulgin, who first synthesized the drug in 1965; therapists found that it proved an effective form of treatment for marriage, counselling, PTSD, stress, depression and schizophrenia (Griffin, 2012).

However despite the evidence from those in therapeutic practice of the benefits of ecstasy use as a treatment intervention there is evidence that appears to suggest that MDMA is associated with psychological mental health issues. The literature on MDMA and psychological deficits are linked to numerous psychiatric problems/ psychobiological problems including depression, obsessive-compulsive disorder, paranoia, poor appetite and altered sleep (McCardle et al, 2004). These researchers have argued for health interventions by professionals, and a change in legal policy in promotion of illegalization of drugs. Furthermore there is increasing literature linking ecstasy to problems/ deficits with the central executive component of memory (Hanson et al, 2010). Some of those investigating MDMA neurological affects argue there is a case/ argument that MDMA can cause neurodegenerative problems with the brain and affect the psychobiology of the brain in a negative, damaging and dangerous way (Mohamed et al, 2011; Parrot, 2013a, 2014). However, the research must be viewed critically since it is currently unclear whether the patients have pre-existing mental health problems prior to ecstasy use; therefore no evidence of psychological damage can be attributed to MDMA use primarily (Guillot et al, 2007). The evidence of cross-sectional studies suggests that psychiatric symptoms appear before the onset of ecstasy use, rather than as a direct result of the use of the substance (Guillot et al, 2007). Lieb et al. (2002) found that 88% of ecstasy users diagnosed with a mental health disorder had the disorder prior to use of MDMA. This was a significant study indicating a need for future studies on those who have not been previously diagnosed in order to validate Lieb et al. (2002) findings. In support of the cross-sectional studies conducted there appears to be strong evidence from longitudinal studies which have failed to identify any psychiatric symptoms caused by ecstasy use (Guillot et al, 2007). Win et al. (2006) conducted a longitudinal study of two years on ecstasy users and found no evidence for mental health conditions concerning depression, sensation-seeking and impulsivity levels across the time-span. Thomasius et al. (2005) conducted a cross-sectional study which showed that the drug-user group was three times more likely to have life-long attention deficit/hyperactivity disorder (ADHD) in comparison to the drug-naïve control group. These findings suggest that mental health problems may be a significant risk factor to pre-substance drug-taking, but do not apply to the effects of MDMA in isolation on the brain structure. There also appears to be a strong methodological limitation to these studies since some have not conducted psychiatric assessments prior to the study, and also may not have assessed whether the participant is using a multitude of different drugs with their own effects. This complicates findings and conclusions since any attempt to apply negative psychological conclusions is reductive in light of MDMA users who are likely to use other drugs in conjunction with ecstasy (Hanson et al, 2010). The methodological limitation is that conducting tests and experiments on participants who have only used, or using MDMA in isolation are hard to obtain with any cognitive or psychological deficits hard to accurately explain due to the high rate of comorbid drug use.

Furthermore there is a strong overlap with drug researchers and politics due to the legal policy status of certain drugs and there personal and medical uses. The cost to society approach is often used by prohibitionists who state the cost of drug abuse on the National Health Service (NHS) and business productivity decline due to substance abuse (Caulkins et al, 2014). The current debate between Parrott et al. (2013; 2014) and Doblin et al. (2014) is of significant interest in examining the existing state of MDMA research in the past 25 years. Parrott (2013a) in his analysis of the studies conducted on MDMA use and effects in the past twenty five years concluded that MDMA is now in a position where it should be viewed as a 'dangerous' drug. This however, has several major flaws which Doblin et al. (2014) seeks to remedy. Firstly Parrott (2013a) often focuses on the use of recreational studies which have indicated reduced cognitive processing, memory loss and recall deficits in all areas except visual memory, and 5HT (serotonin) withdrawal temporarily after the come down, or hangover effect of the drug (Colado et al, 2004; Zakzanis and Young, 2006; Roberts et al, 2009; Benningfield and Cowan, 2013). However, there are several methodological limitations to this argument. Firstly there appears to be a lack of distinction between medical psychotherapy in a supervised experiment with pure MDMA; and recreational use with numerous polydrug users, unsupervised environments and ecstasy which has a high probability of not being pure MDMA but a mixture of other illicit substances (Hayner, 2002; Meyer, 2013). Therefore studies that are case studies or cross-sectional have to be treated with caution in light of their findings since there are serious methodological limitations with large numbers of ecstasy users fitting the criteria of polydrug users; those who use other substances alongside MDMA. Furthermore (Parrott, 2014) in his rebuttal to Doblin et al's (2013) criticisms suggests that psychotherapy benefits may apply to a number of individuals but it can be 'counter-productive' in others. There is absolutely no modern empirical evidence for this assertion, the only evidence that Parrott cites is from the anecdotal report conducted by Greer and Tolbert (1986) where one elderly individual reported some negative side-effects related to insomnia, loss of appetite and blurred vision. The conclusion that MDMA is therefore not wise to use in psychotherapy settings is drastically ill-informed, with little empirical support and suggests that Parrott has allowed emotions and fear-driven scenarios to cloud scientific objectivity and understanding. This fear and inability to explore the therapeutic benefits by some drug researchers is hindering progress and scientific objectivity to establish equal sides of the argument and concentrating research on establishing conclusions primarily on recreational users and polydrug users. What is needed is for decriminalization to open up the doorway to large sample size, longitudinal studies that investigate effects of MDMA doses over periods of time with fluctuating dose sample sizes (Mithoefer, 2011).

The biological evidence has identified several key factors that are ubiquitously accepted by those in scientific investigation of the effects of MDMA on neuroplasticity and brain structure. The drug has been investigated to have a strong connection with 5-HT, serotonin release into the neural pathways and serotonin receptor 2 stimulation (Green et al, 2003; Gudelsky et al, 2008; Schenk, 2011; White, 2014). The evidence suggests that this serotonin agonist response is the cause of increased empathetic skills and positive relationships that are a result of MDMA properties; particularly the serotonin effect on the oxytocin levels which influence pro-social behaviours either directly or indirectly, and reduce negative emotions towards others (Mithoefer, 2011; Meyer, 2013). There also appears to be higher levels of prolactin and cortisol. Cortisol is increasingly shown to be linked to the stress response; this may explain those who have stated elevated levels of stress and fear during ecstasy use. Mithoefer (2011) study found that an elevation in oxytocin levels was linked to an increase in cerebral blood flow 75 minutes after MDMA administration in healthy volunteers. It was found that cerebral blood flow increased in the ventromedial frontal and occipital cortex, with reduced blood levels in the amygdala. The amygdala is associated with memory; in relation to therapeutic benefits this may explain why MDMA has demonstrated its potentials as an effective intervention tool in treating those with posttraumatic stress disorder; at least during the time that the effects are in swing during the first six hours of administration of the drug (Smith, 2007; White, 2014). Beck and Rosenbaum (1994) phenomenological study: reported that there are two types of MDMA users; the therapeutic user and the recreational user. The therapeutic user in studies of MDMA have not reported any significance of addiction to MDMA, they are able to discontinue use of the drug with little sign of dependence on ecstasy use (Peroutka, 1990) it seldom accompanies ecstasy use unlike heroin or cocaine (Agar et al, 2004). In addition there appears to be little evidence for some of the negative effects that have been found in illicit drug taking of recreational settings. The two most common negative physiological effects appear to be hyperthermia and dehydration; however in a controlled medical setting these are unlikely to occur (Mithoefer, 2011). There have been attempts to link ecstasy use with dependence, however many are based on case studies with a small collection of individuals. For instance, Jansen (1999) argued that MDMA had been shown to demonstrate dependent behaviours on the drug from three case studies outlining their life background and how ecstasy use had been involved. In each case however, they were using other substances such as cannabis, amphetamine, heroin and benzodiazepine. These findings cannot be applied to scientific enquiry into MDMA use since they are polydrug users, with most users using multiple forms of substances (Hanson, 2010).

The main methodological limitation is that large scale, longitudinal studies with long-term drug administration is currently unethical under current legal restrictions (Smith, 2007; Sessa and Nutt, 2007; Mithoefer, 2011; Caulkins et al, 2014). The role of criminalization has been to severely stunt the scientific community from investigating illicit drugs such as MDMA in a controlled, medical environment. This research is needed however to expand and develop upon the anecdotal reports that therapists conducted in the 1970s and early 1980s into therapeutic benefits before the decision issued by the DEA to classify MDMA as a Schedule 1 substance, and the United Kingdom's decision to label MDMA as a Class A, schedule 1 drug (Sessa and Nutt, 2007). The UK needs to adopt a decriminalization system that is akin to its neighbouring European neighbours such as Portugal. There has been no major surge in drug use, as predicted by the prohibitionists, and they have successfully implemented a medical/health model where recreational drugs such as MDMA can be applied and referred to patients based on a professional and clinical assessment; evidence suggests that it operates as an effective treatment tool for PTSD (Smith, 2007). Furthermore since the link between social integration and MDMA use has been established, it would prove an effective method of treating anxiety disorders where the person is incapable of disclosure and social exploration. This recommendation and legislative change would lead to further studies investigating the effects of MDMA over longer periods of time, with differing doses. The positive effects of MDMA: the sense of euphoria, increased sex drive, social integration and strong wish to socialize with people (Wardle, 2014). These are all aspects which have been hindered by legislative restrictions and have stunted future scientific investigation into the therapeutic benefits of MDMA; there has been very little progress with severely limited strong, empirical, longitudinal research into the effects of MDMA since the criminalization process in the 1980s, but there is evidence that clinical research into MDMA is gaining momentum (Mithoefer, 2011). However, most empirical research into the biological neurology of MDMA use has been confined to animal studies, particularly rats and their behaviour. These of course have reduced the empirical validity of the conclusions into MDMA; there needs to be further human trials conducted, longitudinal in design, with varying degrees of dosage administered. The social harm that is currently caused by criminalization measures is also gravely concerning, research indicates that those in possession of drugs are increasingly issued with criminal records for possession of drugs such as cannabis and MDMA. These are correlated with long-term drug addiction, unemployment, lack of social aspirations. These exacerbate the underlying drug addiction and cause deterioration in socio-economic status. Furthermore the resources of the Criminal Prosecution Service are increasingly strained when it could be dealing with more severe cases in the criminal justice system (Smith, 2007; Ward, 2013).

References

Agar, M & Reisinger, H. S. (2004). Ecstasy: Commodity or disease? *Journal of Psychoactive Drugs*, 36(2), 253-264.

Beck, J., & Rosenbaum, M. (1994). Pursuit of ecstasy: The MDMA experience. Albany, NY: State University of New York Press.

Caulkins, J. P., Kasunic, A., Kleiman, M., & Lee, M. (2014). Understanding drug legalization. *International Public Health Journal*, 6(3), 283-294.

Clegg, N., & Branson, R. (21st May 2015). We have been losing the war on drugs for decades for four decades-end it now. *The Guardian*, 1-3.

Colado, M.I., O'Shea, E., Green, A.R. (2004). Acute and long-term effects of MDMA on cerebral dopamine biochemistry and function, *Psychopharmacology*, 173, 249-263.

Doblin, R., Greer, G., Holland, J., Jerome, L., Mithoefer, M.C., & Sessa, B. (2014). A reconsideration and response to Parrott AC (2013) "Human psychobiology of MDMA or "ecstasy": an overview of 25 years of empirical research. *Human Psychopharmacology Clinical Experience*, 29, 105-108.

Greer, G.R., Tolbert, R. (1986). Subjective reports of the effects of MDMA in a clinical setting. *Journal of Psychoactive Drugs*, 18(4), 319-327.

Griffin O.H. (2012). Is the government keeping the peace or acting like our parents? Rationales for the legal prohibitions of GBH and MDMA. *Journal of Drug Issues*, 42(3), 247-262.

Guillot, C.R., & Berman, M.E. (2007). MDMA (Ecstasy) use and psychiatric problems. *Psychopharmacology*, 189, 575-576.

Hanson, K.L., Luciana, M. (2010). Neurocognitive impairments in MDMA and other drug users: MDMA alone may not be a cognitive risk factor. *Journal of Clinical and Experimental Neuropsychology*. 32(4), 337-349.

Hayner, G.N. (2002). MDMA misrepresentation: An unresolved problem for ecstasy users. *Journal of Psychoactive Drugs*, 34(2), 195-198.

Jansen, K.LR. (1999). Ecstasy (MDMA) dependence. *Drug and Alcohol Dependence*, 53, 121-124.

Lieb, R., Schuetz, C., Pfister, H., Von Skydow, K., & Wittchen, H. (2002). Mental disorders in ecstasy users: a prospective-longitudinal investigation. *Drug and Alcohol Dependence*, 68(2), 195.

Meyer, J.S. (2013). 3,4-methlenedioxymethamphetamine (MDMA): current perspectives. *Substance abuse and rehabilitation*, 4, 83-99.

Mithoefer, M.C. (2011). Does MDMA have a role in clinical psychiatry? *Psychiatric Times*, 36-49.

Mohamed, W.M.Y., Hamida, S.B., Cassel, J.C., Vasconcelos, A.P.D., & Jones. C.B. (2011). MDMA: Interactions with other psychoactive drugs. *Pharmacology, Biochemistry and Behavior*, 99, 759-774.

Parrott, A.C. (2001). Human psychopharmacology of Ecstasy (MDMA): A review of 15 years of empirical research. *Human Psychopharmacology*, 16, 557-77.

Parrott, A.C. (2014). MDMA is certainly damaging after 25 years of empirical research: a reply and refutation of Doblin et al. (2014). *Human Psychopharmacology*, 29, 109-119.

Peroutka, S.J. (1990). Recreational use of MDMA. *Human Psychopharmacology*, 53-63.

Roberts, G.M., Nestor, L., Garavan, H. (2009). Learning and memory deficits in ecstasy users and their natural correlates during a face-learning task. *Brain Research*, 1292, 71-87.

Schenk, S. (2011). MDMA ("ecstasy") abuse as an example of dopamine neuroplasticity. *Neuroscience and Biobehavioural Reviews*, 35, 1203-1218.

Sessa, B., & Nutt, D. J. (2007). MDMA, politics and medical research: Have we thrown the baby out with the bathwater? *Journal of Psychopharmacology*, 21(8), 787-791.

Smith, J. (2007). Values and control of MDMA. *Contemporary Justice Review: Issues in Criminal, Social and Restorative Justice.* 10(3), 297-306.

Thomasius, R., Petersen, K.U., Zapletalova, P., Wartberg, L., Zeichner, D., & Schmoldt, A. (2005). Mental disorders in current and former heavy ecstasy (MDMA) users. *Addiction.* 100, 1310-1319.

Ward, J. (2013). Punishing drug possession in the magistrates' courts: time for a rethink. *European Journal of Criminal Policy*, 19, 289-307.

Wardle, M.C., Wit, H.D. (2014). MDMA alters emotional processing and facilitates positive social interaction. *Psychopharmacology*, 231, 4219-4229.

White, M.C. (2014). 3,4- Methylenedioxymethamphetamine's (MDMA's) Impact on Posttraumatic Stress Disorder. *Annals of Pharmacotherapy*, 48(7), 908-915.

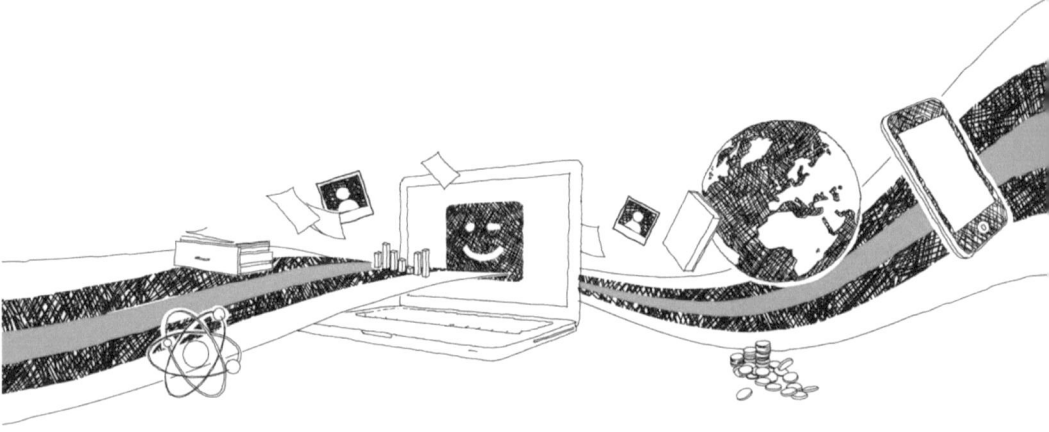
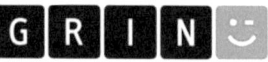